SYMPTOMS OF KIDNEY DISEASE

UNDERSTANDING SYMPTOMS OF KIDNEY DISEASE

Estefan Giovanni

TABLE OF CONTENT

INTRODUCTION

INTRODUCTION TO KIDNEY DISEASE AND ITS PREVALENCE

Introduction to Kidney Disease and Its Prevalence

The human body's intricate network of organs and systems relies on a delicate balance to maintain optimal health. Among the unsung heroes of this equilibrium are the kidneys, two bean-shaped organs located on either side of the spine. While often underestimated, the kidneys play a vital role in filtering waste, regulating fluid and electrolyte levels, and supporting overall well-being. However, this essential function isn't always safeguarded. Kidney disease, a condition that impairs the kidneys' ability to perform their tasks effectively, poses a significant threat to health.

Kidney disease can range from minor functional disruptions to severe disorders with potentially life-threatening consequences. As we delve into the intricate world of kidney health, it becomes evident that understanding kidney disease's symptoms and implications is crucial for maintaining a high quality of life.

PREVALENCE OF KIDNEY DISEASE: A GROWING CONCERN

In recent years, kidney disease has emerged as a global health concern, affecting millions of individuals regardless of age, gender, or ethnicity. According to the World Health Organization (WHO), kidney disease ranks as the 12th leading cause of death worldwide. The prevalence of kidney disease is amplified by its close connections to other chronic conditions, such as diabetes and hypertension. Chronic Kidney Disease (CKD), a common form of kidney disease, is particularly noteworthy due to its increasing prevalence. The Centers for Disease Control and Prevention (CDC) estimate that around 15% of adults in the United States have CKD. This statistic is alarming not only because of the disease's direct impact on kidney function but also due to its association with a heightened risk of heart disease and stroke.

THE SILENT THREAT: IMPORTANCE OF EARLY DETECTION

One of the challenges of kidney disease lies in its often subtle and insidious nature. In the early stages, symptoms might be vague or easily mistaken for other health issues, leading to delayed diagnosis and treatment. However, the consequences of neglecting kidney health can be severe, potentially leading to irreversible damage and a reduced quality of life. The silver lining is that early detection of kidney disease can be a game-changer. Recognizing the symptoms and risk factors allows individuals to take proactive steps towards managing the condition, slowing its progression, and minimizing complications. This is where understanding the symptoms of kidney disease becomes pivotal—enabling individuals, healthcare providers, and communities to collaborate effectively in the pursuit of better kidney health.

EMBARKING ON A JOURNEY OF KNOWLEDGE

As we embark on this journey to unravel the intricacies of kidney disease and its symptoms, we will explore the various types of kidney diseases, delve into the diverse array of symptoms they can manifest, and equip ourselves with the knowledge needed to advocate for our own health and the health of those around us. By shedding light on kidney disease and its prevalence, we aim to empower individuals to take an active role in safeguarding their kidney health and, by extension, their overall well-being.

THE SIGNIFICANCE OF RECOGNIZING AND UNDERSTANDING SYMPTOMS FOR EARLY DETECTION AND MANAGEMENT OF KIDNEY DISEASE

In the realm of healthcare, knowledge truly is power. When it comes to kidney disease, recognizing and understanding its symptoms can be the difference between timely intervention and irreversible damage. The journey from subtle symptoms to full-blown kidney dysfunction is often a slow, silent progression. However, by familiarizing ourselves with the signs, we can unlock the potential for early detection and effective management, thereby preserving our well-being and quality of life.

TIMELY INTERVENTION SAVES LIVES

Kidney disease is notorious for its ability to lurk beneath the surface, showing minimal signs until it reaches advanced stages. By the time overt symptoms manifest, irreversible damage might already be underway. However, by recognizing even the subtlest changes, individuals can prompt medical evaluation. Early diagnosis opens doors to proactive treatment, lifestyle adjustments, and potential interventions that can slow or even halt the progression of the disease.

Navigating the Web of Symptoms

The symptoms of kidney disease can be varied and sometimes nonspecific, often overlapping with those of other conditions. This complexity can make diagnosis challenging. By understanding the spectrum of symptoms associated with kidney disease—ranging from urinary abnormalities and fluid imbalances to fatigue and cardiovascular complications—we empower ourselves to connect the dots and present a comprehensive picture to healthcare providers. This informed approach expedites accurate diagnosis and personalized treatment plans.

Quality of Life Preservation

The kidneys are integral to maintaining the body's internal equilibrium. Kidney dysfunction can disrupt this balance, leading to a cascade of health issues. Recognizing symptoms early allows for interventions that can mitigate or prevent complications like high blood pressure, electrolyte imbalances, anemia, and bone problems. By preserving these delicate balances, individuals can sustain their energy levels, vitality, and overall quality of life.

Empowerment through Proactive Care

By being attuned to changes in urine color, frequency, or consistency, and by recognizing signs like persistent fatigue, swelling, or unexplained changes in blood pressure, individuals can engage in informed conversations with healthcare providers. This collaborative approach facilitates timely screenings, tests, and personalized strategies for managing kidncy health.

Reduced Healthcare Burden

Late-stage kidney disease often necessitates more intensive and costly interventions, such as dialysis or kidney transplantation. Early detection and management can help avoid these advanced stages, thus reducing the burden on the healthcare system and the financial strain on individuals and families.

Spreading Awareness:

Understanding the significance of recognizing symptoms extends beyond individual well-being. By raising awareness about kidney disease symptoms and their implications, we contribute to a more informed society that prioritizes kidney health. This collective knowledge helps reduce the stigma associated with kidney disease and encourages regular health check-ups, benefiting communities at large.

CHAPTER 1: THE BASICS OF KIDNEY FUNCTION

EXPLANATION OF THE KIDNEYS' PRIMARY ROLES: FILTRATION, WASTE REMOVAL, FLUID BALANCE, ELECTROLYTE REGULATION

The kidneys are remarkable organs that perform a multitude of essential functions crucial for maintaining the body's overall health and equilibrium. Their intricate roles can be broadly categorized into four primary functions: filtration, waste removal, fluid balance, and electrolyte regulation.

Filtration:

Filtration is one of the kidneys' fundamental functions. Each kidney is composed of numerous microscopic structures called nephrons. These nephrons are responsible for filtering the blood to remove waste products, excess substances, and toxins. The process begins with blood entering the kidneys through specialized blood vessels called glomeruli. In the glomeruli, blood pressure forces small molecules, such as water, electrolytes, and waste products, to pass through tiny filtration barriers while retaining larger molecules like proteins and blood cells. This filtered fluid, known as filtrate, moves into the renal tubules for further processing.

Waste Removal:

Once the filtrate enters the renal tubules, the kidneys meticulously regulate the composition of this fluid. Unwanted waste products, such as urea, creatinine, and excess ions, are actively removed from the filtrate and transported into the tubules. These waste products would otherwise accumulate in the bloodstream, potentially leading to harmful effects on various body systems. The kidneys' ability to efficiently eliminate waste ensures that the body remains free from the toxic byproducts of metabolism.

Fluid Balance:

Maintaining the body's fluid balance is another critical role of the kidneys. By selectively reabsorbing water and essential ions from the filtrate as it travels through the renal tubules, the kidneys help regulate the body's overall fluid volume. When the body is dehydrated, the kidneys prioritize water reabsorption to conserve fluid and prevent excessive loss. Conversely, during periods of excess fluid intake, the kidneys excrete surplus water through urine to maintain the body's optimal hydration levels.

Electrolyte Regulation:

Electrolytes are electrically charged ions that play pivotal roles in various bodily functions, including nerve transmission, muscle contraction, and pH regulation. The kidneys are responsible for fine-tuning the concentrations of electrolytes like sodium, potassium, calcium, and phosphate in the bloodstream. Through processes such as selective reabsorption and secretion, the kidneys ensure that these electrolyte levels remain within narrow ranges to support proper physiological functioning.

IMPORTANCE OF MAINTAINING KIDNEY HEALTH FOR OVERALL WELL-BEING

Maintaining kidney health is not only essential for the proper functioning of the kidneys themselves but also plays a crucial role in ensuring overall well-being and the optimal functioning of the entire body. The kidneys are intricately connected to various physiological processes, and their health impacts multiple systems.

Waste Removal and Detoxification:

The kidneys act as the body's natural filtration system, removing waste products, toxins, and excess substances from the bloodstream. If the kidneys aren't functioning properly, these waste products can accumulate, leading to a buildup of harmful substances that can negatively impact various organs and systems. Maintaining healthy kidneys ensures efficient waste removal and detoxification, supporting the body's overall metabolic processes.

Fluid and Electrolyte Balance:

Healthy kidneys are responsible for maintaining a delicate balance of fluids and electrolytes in the body. Proper fluid balance is essential for maintaining blood pressure, regulating body temperature, and supporting cellular functions. Imbalances can lead to issues such as dehydration, electrolyte disorders, and hypertension, which can have far-reaching effects on overall health.

Blood Pressure Regulation:

They help control blood pressure by adjusting the volume of blood in circulation and releasing hormones that influence blood vessel constriction and dilation. When kidney function is compromised, blood pressure regulation can be disrupted, potentially leading to hypertension, a major risk factor for cardiovascular diseases.

Red Blood Cell Production:

Red blood cells carry oxygen to tissues and organs, supporting energy production and overall vitality. If kidney function is impaired, the production of erythropoietin can be reduced, leading to anemia and decreased oxygen delivery to cells.

Bone Health:

Kidneys help regulate calcium and phosphorus levels in the blood, which are crucial for bone health. Proper kidney function prevents imbalances that could lead to bone disorders like osteoporosis or bone fractures.

Acid-Base Balance:

Kidneys play a role in maintaining the body's acid-base balance, also known as pH balance. They help eliminate excess acid or base from the body to prevent the blood from becoming too acidic or alkaline. Imbalances in pH can disrupt cellular functions and lead to various health issues.

Metabolic Health:

Kidneys are involved in glucose metabolism, and they help filter glucose from the bloodstream. In conditions like diabetes, the kidneys may be under increased strain, potentially leading to kidney damage. Maintaining kidney health is crucial for managing metabolic disorders and preventing complications.

CHAPTER 2: COMMON TYPES OF KIDNEY DISEASES

BRIEF OVERVIEW OF DIFFERENT TYPES OF KIDNEY DISEASES: CHRONIC KIDNEY DISEASE (CKD), ACUTE KIDNEY INJURY (AKI), POLYCYSTIC KIDNEY DISEASE (PKD), GLOMERULONEPHRITIS

Chronic Kidney Disease (CKD):

CKD is a progressive condition where the kidneys gradually lose their function over time. It is often a result of conditions like diabetes, hypertension, or certain autoimmune diseases. As the kidneys' filtering ability diminishes, waste and fluids can accumulate in the body, leading to various complications. CKD is categorized into stages based on the severity of kidney damage and reduced function.

Acute Kidney Injury (AKI):

AKI, also known as acute renal failure, is a sudden and rapid decline in kidney function. It can be caused by various factors such as severe infections, dehydration, medication side effects, or injury. AKI can lead to a sudden accumulation of waste and fluids in the body, and if not treated promptly, it can be life-threatening.

Polycystic Kidney Disease (PKD):

These cysts can gradually replace healthy kidney tissue, impairing kidney function. PKD can lead to hypertension, chronic pain, and eventually, kidney failure.

Glomerulonephritis:

Glomerulonephritis refers to a group of diseases that primarily affect the glomeruli, which are tiny blood vessels in the kidneys responsible for filtering waste and excess fluids. Inflammation of the glomeruli can impair their filtering function, leading to proteinuria (protein in urine), blood in urine, and reduced kidney function.

Glomerulonephritis can be caused by infections, immune system disorders, or certain medications.

Kidney Stones:

Kidney stones are solid mineral and salt deposits that form within the kidneys. They can be painful and cause symptoms such as severe flank pain, blood in urine, and difficulty urinating. Kidney stones vary in size and can block the urinary tract, leading to complications if not managed properly.

Kidney Infections (Pyelonephritis):

A kidney infection is a bacterial infection that affects one or both kidneys. It typically starts as a urinary tract infection and can spread to the kidneys. Symptoms include fever, back pain, frequent urination, and cloudy or bloody urine. If left untreated, kidney infections can cause damage to the kidneys and lead to sepsis.

Chronic Kidney Disease (CKD):

Causes: CKD often develops as a result of long-term conditions that damage the kidneys' structures and impair their function. Common underlying causes include diabetes, hypertension (high blood pressure), glomerulonephritis, and polycystic kidney disease.

Risk Factors: Risk factors for CKD include diabetes, hypertension, family history of kidney disease, older age, obesity, smoking, and certain ethnic backgrounds (such as African American, Hispanic, Native American).

Acute Kidney Injury (AKI):

Causes: AKI is usually triggered by sudden and severe conditions that disrupt blood flow to the kidneys or directly damage kidney tissues. Common causes include dehydration, severe infections (sepsis), certain medications (such as nonsteroidal anti-inflammatory drugs or NSAIDs), and conditions that obstruct the urinary tract.

Polycystic Kidney Disease (PKD):

Causes: PKD is a genetic disorder caused by mutations in certain genes. These mutations lead to the development of fluid-filled cysts in the kidneys, which gradually replace normal kidney tissue.

Glomerulonephritis:

Causes: Glomerulonephritis is often the result of an immune system response that leads to inflammation and damage to the glomeruli, the kidney's filtering units. It can be triggered by infections (such as streptococcal infections), immune system disorders (such as lupus), or other underlying conditions.

CHAPTER 3: RECOGNIZING THE RED FLAGS: GENERAL SYMPTOMS

DISCUSSION OF COMMON EARLY-STAGE SYMPTOMS: FATIGUE, FREQUENT URINATION, CHANGES IN URINE COLOR AND VOLUME.

COMMON EARLY-STAGE SYMPTOMS OF KIDNEY DISEASE

Early-stage kidney disease can often present with subtle and nonspecific symptoms, which may be mistaken for other health issues. Recognizing these symptoms is crucial for timely intervention and management.

Fatigue

Feeling unusually tired or fatigued is a common early symptom of kidney disease. This can occur due to the kidneys' reduced ability to filter waste products and toxins from the blood, leading to a buildup of waste in the body. Additionally, anemia, which often accompanies kidney disease, can contribute to fatigue. Anemia occurs when the kidneys produce less erythropoietin, a hormone that stimulates red blood cell production.

Frequent Urination:

An increase in the frequency of urination, especially at night (nocturia), can be an early sign of kidney dysfunction. The kidneys play a role in regulating fluid balance, and when they aren't functioning properly, excess fluids can accumulate in the body.

Changes in Urine Color and Volume:

Changes in urine color and volume can provide valuable insights into kidney health. Darker urine than usual, or blood in the urine (hematuria), may indicate damage to the kidneys' filtering units or urinary tract. Foamy or frothy urine might suggest excess protein in the urine, which can be a sign of impaired kidney function. Changes in urine volume, such as producing more or less urine than usual, can also indicate kidney-related issues.

Kidney problems can indeed lead to anemia due to their role in producing a hormone called erythropoietin (EPO). Erythropoietin plays a crucial role in stimulating the production of red blood cells in the bone marrow. When kidney function is compromised, the production of EPO can decrease, resulting in a condition known as "anemia of chronic kidney disease" or "renal anemia." This condition can have a significant impact on the body and manifest through various associated symptoms.

HOW KIDNEY PROBLEMS CAUSE ANEMIA

EPO Production Reduction: In healthy individuals, the kidneys detect the levels of oxygen in the blood and release erythropoietin in response to low oxygen levels. EPO travels to the bone marrow, where it stimulates the production of red blood cells, which carry oxygen to tissues. In kidney disease, the damaged kidneys may produce less EPO, leading to decreased red blood cell production.

Shortened Red Blood Cell Lifespan: Kidney disease can also result in the accumulation of waste products and toxins in the blood. These substances can affect the lifespan of red blood cells, causing them to break down more quickly than usual, contributing to anemia.

Associated Symptoms of Anemia in Kidney Disease

Fatigue and Weakness: Anemia reduces the amount of oxygen delivered to body tissues. This can lead to feelings of fatigue, weakness, and decreased stamina. Even simple activities can become exhausting.

Pale Skin and Nail Beds: Due to decreased oxygen supply, individuals with anemia often have pale skin and nail beds. The reduced oxygen levels can also lead to a bluish tint in the lips and fingertips (cyanosis).

Shortness of Breath: Anemia can cause the heart to work harder to compensate for the reduced oxygen-carrying capacity of the blood.

Dizziness and Headache: Reduced oxygen supply to the brain can cause dizziness, lightheadedness, and headaches.

Cold Sensitivity: Anemia can lead to poor circulation, causing some individuals to feel cold more easily.

Cognitive Impairment: In severe cases, anemia can affect cognitive function, leading to difficulty concentrating, memory problems, and overall cognitive impairment.

Irregular Heartbeat: Anemia can strain the cardiovascular system, leading to an irregular heartbeat (arrhythmia) and worsening hypertension.

THE CONNECTION BETWEEN KIDNEY HEALTH AND BONE HEALTH, AND RELATED SYMPTOMS

The connection between kidney health and bone health is intricate and essential, primarily due to the kidneys' role in maintaining proper levels of calcium and phosphorus in the body. When kidney function is compromised, it can lead to imbalances in these minerals, which in turn can negatively affect bone health. This connection is particularly important because healthy bones provide structural support, protect vital organs, and store minerals that contribute to various physiological processes.

KIDNEY HEALTH'S IMPACT ON BONE HEALTH

Calcium and Phosphorus Regulation: The kidneys play a crucial role in regulating calcium and phosphorus levels in the blood. Proper calcium levels are essential for bone mineralization, while phosphorus is also a critical component of bone structure. Kidneys activate vitamin D, which enhances calcium absorption in the intestines. When kidney function declines, calcium absorption and phosphorus excretion can be disrupted, leading to imbalances.

Parathyroid Hormone (PTH) Regulation: The parathyroid glands, located near the thyroid gland, secrete parathyroid hormone (PTH) in response to low blood calcium levels. PTH helps regulate calcium and phosphorus by stimulating their release from bones and enhancing their absorption from the intestines. In kidney disease, abnormal PTH levels can result in bone resorption (loss of bone density), weakening bones over time.

IMPACT ON BONE HEALTH AND SYMPTOMS:

Bone Fractures: Imbalances in calcium and phosphorus levels, along with weakened bone structure, increase the risk of bone fractures. Individuals with kidney disease, particularly those with abnormal mineral metabolism, are more susceptible to fractures, even with minor trauma.

Bone Pain: Calcium imbalances can lead to bone pain. Individuals may experience dull, aching bone pain, especially in the back and joints. This pain can affect mobility and overall quality of life.

Osteoporosis: Long-term kidney disease, particularly chronic kidney disease (CKD), can contribute to a condition known as renal osteodystrophy. This term encompasses a range of bone disorders that can lead to osteoporosis, bone pain, and an increased risk of fractures.

Bone Deformities: Imbalances in calcium and phosphorus can result in bone deformities, particularly in children with kidney disease. This condition is known as renal rickets and can affect growth and bone development.

Hyperparathyroidism: In kidney disease, an imbalance in calcium, phosphorus, and vitamin D can lead to overactive parathyroid glands. This condition, called secondary hyperparathyroidism, can result in bone resorption, bone pain, and an increased risk of fractures.

CHAPTER 4: URINARY ABNORMALITIES

DETAILED DESCRIPTION OF URINARY SYMPTOMS: CHANGES IN FREQUENCY, URGENCY, AND CONSISTENCY OF URINE

Urinary symptoms are often early indicators of various health issues, including kidney and urinary tract problems. Changes in the frequency, urgency, and consistency of urine can provide valuable insights into underlying conditions.

Changes in Frequency:

Increased Frequency (Polyuria): This refers to an increased need to urinate more often than usual. It can be caused by factors such as excessive fluid intake, diabetes (which leads to increased urine output due to high blood sugar levels), urinary tract infections (UTIs), and certain medications. In kidney disease, reduced kidney function can lead to decreased urine concentration, causing increased urine production and frequency.

Decreased Frequency (Oliguria): Oliguria is characterized by producing less urine than usual. It can result from dehydration, urinary tract obstructions (such as kidney stones or enlarged prostate), kidney disease, or acute kidney injury (AKI). Decreased urine output can be a concerning sign, especially if accompanied by other symptoms like swelling, fatigue, and changes in urine color.

Urgency:

Urgency refers to a sudden and compelling need to urinate. It can be a normal response when the bladder is full, but persistent urgency that's not relieved by urination might be indicative of conditions such as overactive bladder, urinary tract infections, or neurological issues affecting bladder control. Kidney stones or infections that irritate the urinary tract can also cause urgency.

Consistency of Urine:

Foamy or Frothy Urine: Excess protein in the urine can cause it to appear foamy or frothy. Proteinuria (presence of protein in urine) can be a sign of

kidney disease, particularly when the kidneys'
filtering units are damaged. It's important to have
proteinuria evaluated by a healthcare professional,
as it can indicate underlying kidney issues.

Blood in Urine (Hematuria): Hematuria refers to
the presence of blood in the urine, which can give
the urine a pink, red, or brownish color. Hematuria
can occur due to infections, kidney stones, urinary
tract injuries, and various kidney diseases. It's
crucial to have hematuria assessed, as it can
indicate conditions that need prompt medical
attention.

Cloudy or Murky Urine: Cloudy urine can result
from various factors, including infections (such as
UTIs), kidney stones, and excess crystals in the
urine. Cloudiness can also be due to high levels of
white blood cells or bacteria.

Strong Odor: Unusual or strong-smelling urine can
be caused by dehydration, certain foods,
medications, or urinary tract infections. In some

cases, kidney-related issues can contribute to changes in urine odor.

EXPLORATION OF FOAMY URINE, ITS POSSIBLE CAUSES, AND ITS LINK TO KIDNEY DISEASE

Foamy urine, also known as proteinuria or bubbly urine, refers to urine that has an excessive amount of bubbles or foam when it's passed. While it's normal for urine to have some bubbles due to the force of urination, persistent foamy urine can be a sign of an underlying issue, including kidney-related problems. Let's explore the possible causes of foamy urine and its link to kidney disease:

POSSIBLE CAUSES OF FOAMY URINE:

Proteinuria: One of the primary causes of foamy urine is the presence of excess protein in the urine, a condition known as proteinuria. Healthy kidneys filter waste products from the blood while keeping essential proteins in the bloodstream. When the kidneys' filtering units (glomeruli) are damaged, they may allow proteins to pass into the urine. This excess protein can create bubbles and cause urine to appear foamy.

Dehydration: Dehydration can cause the urine to become more concentrated, leading to increased foaming. When there's insufficient water intake, urine can contain higher levels of waste products, which can result in foamy appearance.

Urinary Tract Infections (UTIs): UTIs can irritate the urinary tract, leading to increased production of mucus and other substances that contribute to foam formation in the urine.

Vigorous Urination: Forceful or vigorous urination can introduce air into the urine stream, creating temporary bubbles that cause foamy urine. This is more likely to occur when the bladder is very full.

Foamy urine, particularly if it's persistent, can be a sign of kidney disease or damage. Proteinuria, which is a common cause of foamy urine, can indicate that the kidneys' filtration function is compromised.

Chronic Kidney Disease (CKD): As kidney function declines, the glomeruli's ability to retain proteins becomes impaired, leading to proteinuria. CKD is a progressive condition that can result in significant protein loss in the urine.

Glomerulonephritis: This group of kidney diseases primarily affects the glomeruli, causing inflammation and damage. Proteinuria is a hallmark of glomerulonephritis and can lead to foamy urine.

Diabetic Nephropathy: Diabetes can damage the blood vessels and glomeruli in the kidneys, resulting in proteinuria. Foamy urine may indicate diabetic nephropathy, a common complication of diabetes.

Nephrotic Syndrome: This condition involves a combination of symptoms, including heavy proteinuria, swelling (edema), low blood protein levels, and high cholesterol. Foamy urine is often an early sign of nephrotic syndrome.

HEMATURIA (BLOOD IN URINE) AND ITS POTENTIAL IMPLICATIONS

Hematuria, also known as blood in the urine, occurs when there is visible or microscopic blood present in the urine. It can be a concerning symptom, as it can indicate underlying health issues ranging from minor to potentially serious conditions. Hematuria can be categorized into two types: gross hematuria (visible blood in the urine) and microscopic hematuria (blood that can only be detected under a microscope).

POTENTIAL CAUSES AND IMPLICATIONS:

Urinary Tract Infections (UTIs): UTIs can cause irritation and inflammation of the urinary tract, leading to blood in the urine. While UTIs are generally not life-threatening, they require prompt treatment to prevent the infection from spreading to the kidneys.

Kidney Stones: Kidney stones, small mineral and salt deposits, can cause bleeding when they irritate the urinary tract as they pass. The bleeding can result in blood in the urine, often accompanied by severe pain in the back or abdomen.

Urinary Tract Trauma: Injury to the urinary tract, such as due to accidents or procedures, can cause bleeding and lead to hematuria.

Bladder or Kidney Infections: Infections of the bladder (cystitis) or kidneys (pyelonephritis) can cause inflammation and bleeding in the urinary tract.

Kidney Disease: Hematuria can be a sign of kidney diseases such as glomerulonephritis, where the filtering units of the kidneys become inflamed and damaged.

Bladder or Kidney Stones: Stones can cause irritation and bleeding as they move through the urinary tract.

Enlarged Prostate or Prostate Infections: In men, enlarged prostate or prostate infections (prostatitis) can lead to hematuria.

Cancers: Hematuria can be a symptom of bladder, kidney, or prostate cancers. Although less common, these conditions require thorough evaluation.

Medications or Blood Thinners: Certain medications or blood thinners can increase the risk of bleeding in the urinary tract.

Exercise-Induced Hematuria: Strenuous exercise can sometimes lead to hematuria due to the breakdown of red blood cells in the bloodstream.

WHEN TO SEEK MEDICAL ATTENTION:

It's important to consult a healthcare professional if you notice blood in your urine, even if it's just a small amount or if it's intermittent.

CHAPTER 5: FLUID AND ELECTROLYTE IMBALANCE

EXPLANATION OF THE KIDNEYS' ROLE IN REGULATING FLUID BALANCE AND ELECTROLYTES

The kidneys play a crucial role in maintaining the body's fluid balance and electrolyte levels, which are essential for proper bodily functions and overall health.

FLUID BALANCE REGULATION:

Filtration: The process starts in the nephrons, the functional units of the kidneys. Blood is filtered in tiny blood vessels called glomeruli, where water, electrolytes, and waste products are separated from the blood to form a fluid called filtrate.

Selective Reabsorption: The filtrate then passes through a series of renal tubules, where the kidneys selectively reabsorb water, electrolytes, and important molecules back into the bloodstream. This reabsorption is regulated based on the body's needs to maintain fluid balance.

Antidiuretic Hormone (ADH): When the body senses dehydration or increased blood osmolarity (concentration), the hypothalamus signals the pituitary gland to release ADH. ADH makes the renal tubules more permeable to water, allowing the kidneys to reabsorb more water and concentrate the urine, thereby conserving water.

ELECTROLYTE REGULATION

Sodium (Na+): The kidneys play a central role in regulating sodium levels. Sodium is the most abundant extracellular electrolyte and is vital for maintaining fluid balance, nerve transmission, and muscle function. The kidneys adjust sodium reabsorption in response to factors like blood pressure, hormone levels (such as aldosterone), and overall hydration status.

Potassium (K+): The kidneys control potassium levels by reabsorbing or excreting it. Proper potassium balance is crucial for maintaining proper nerve and muscle function, including the heart. The kidneys adjust potassium excretion based on dietary intake and other factors.

Calcium (Ca2+), Magnesium (Mg2+), and Phosphate (PO4): These electrolytes are also regulated by the kidneys. Calcium is vital for bone health, nerve transmission, and muscle contraction. The kidneys help maintain calcium balance by adjusting its reabsorption and activating vitamin D. Magnesium and phosphate are also involved in various bodily processes.

Acid-Base Balance (pH Regulation): The kidneys play a pivotal role in maintaining the body's acid-base balance. They regulate the levels of hydrogen ions (H+) and bicarbonate ions (HCO3-) in the blood, helping to prevent excessive acidity (acidosis) or alkalinity (alkalosis) in the body.

DISCUSSION OF SYMPTOMS RELATED TO FLUID RETENTION AND EDEMA.

Fluid retention, also known as edema, occurs when excess fluid accumulates in the body's tissues. Edema can be localized, affecting specific areas like the legs or ankles, or it can be generalized, affecting the whole body. Edema can be a sign of various underlying conditions, and recognizing its symptoms is important for proper evaluation and management.

COMMON SYMPTOMS OF EDEMA:

Swelling: Swelling is the hallmark symptom of edema. Affected areas may appear visibly swollen or feel puffy and tight to the touch. Swelling can occur in the ankles, legs, feet, hands, face, or other parts of the body.

Pitting Edema: When pressure is applied to the swollen area, a temporary indentation or "pit" may remain after the pressure is released. This is known as pitting edema and is often used as an indicator of the severity of edema.

Weight Gain: Rapid or unexplained weight gain can be a sign of fluid retention. This weight gain is due to the accumulation of excess fluid in the body's tissues.

Stretched or Shiny Skin: The skin over swollen areas may appear stretched, shiny, or even translucent due to the increased fluid content. This can make the skin more susceptible to tearing and infections.

Discomfort or Pain: Edema can cause discomfort, a feeling of tightness, and even pain in the affected areas. This discomfort can impact mobility and overall quality of life.

Limited Range of Motion: Swelling can restrict the range of motion in joints, making movement more difficult.

POSSIBLE CAUSES AND CONDITIONS ASSOCIATED WITH EDEMA:

Heart Failure: A weakened heart may struggle to pump blood efficiently, leading to fluid backup in the veins and resulting in edema, often in the legs and ankles.

Kidney Disease: Reduced kidney function can lead to fluid and sodium retention, resulting in edema.

Liver Disease: Liver dysfunction can cause changes in blood flow and protein production, contributing to fluid retention.

Venous Insufficiency: Damaged or weakened veins may struggle to return blood to the heart effectively, leading to edema in the legs.

Pregnancy: Hormonal changes and increased pressure on blood vessels during pregnancy can cause fluid retention, particularly in the lower extremities.

Medications: Some medications, such as certain blood pressure drugs or nonsteroidal anti-inflammatory drugs (NSAIDs), can lead to fluid retention as a side effect.

Lymphatic System Issues: Damage or dysfunction of the lymphatic system can impede the proper drainage of fluid from tissues, leading to edema.

Infections: Infections, particularly in the extremities, can cause inflammation and fluid buildup.

ELECTROLYTE IMBALANCE SYMPTOMS, SUCH AS MUSCLE CRAMPS, WEAKNESS, AND IRREGULAR HEARTBEAT

Electrolytes are minerals that carry an electric charge and are essential for various bodily functions, including nerve signaling, muscle contraction, and fluid balance. An imbalance in electrolyte levels, either too high or too low, can lead to a range of symptoms that affect multiple systems in the body.

Muscle Cramps and Weakness:

Low levels of electrolytes like potassium, calcium, and magnesium can lead to muscle cramps and weakness.

Potassium and magnesium, in particular, play a vital role in proper muscle function. Deficiencies can cause muscles to contract excessively and remain in a state of tension, leading to cramps and weakness.

Irregular Heartbeat (Arrhythmia):

Imbalances in electrolytes like potassium, sodium, and calcium can disrupt the normal electrical signaling in the heart, leading to irregular heartbeats or arrhythmias.

Low potassium levels (hypokalemia) can cause heart palpitations, while high potassium levels (hyperkalemia) can lead to dangerous arrhythmias.

Fatigue and Weakness:

Electrolyte imbalances can result in fatigue and overall weakness due to their impact on muscle and nerve function.

Low levels of sodium, for example, can lead to a lack of energy and a feeling of weakness.

Nausea, Vomiting, and Diarrhea:

Electrolyte imbalances, particularly high levels of sodium, can lead to symptoms of nausea, vomiting, and diarrhea.

Diarrhea and vomiting can cause loss of electrolytes and dehydration, which further exacerbates the imbalance.

Confusion and Neurological Symptoms:

Electrolyte imbalances can affect the nervous system, leading to symptoms like confusion, irritability, and changes in mental status.

Low levels of sodium (hyponatremia) can cause neurological symptoms, including confusion and even seizures.

Swelling and Edema:

Electrolyte imbalances, particularly low levels of sodium, can contribute to fluid retention and swelling (edema) in the extremities.

Excessive Thirst and Dry Mouth:

High levels of sodium can lead to dehydration and stimulate excessive thirst and a dry mouth.

CHAPTER 6: BLOOD PRESSURE IRREGULARITIES

UNDERSTANDING THE INTRICATE RELATIONSHIP BETWEEN KIDNEY HEALTH AND BLOOD PRESSURE REGULATION

The intricate relationship between kidney health and blood pressure regulation is of vital importance for maintaining overall physiological balance. The kidneys and blood pressure have a reciprocal relationship, where the kidneys play a significant role in regulating blood pressure, and blood pressure, in turn, affects kidney function. This relationship is crucial for maintaining homeostasis and preventing health issues like hypertension (high blood pressure) and kidney disease.

Renin-Angiotensin-Aldosterone System (RAAS):

The kidneys are central players in the renin-angiotensin-aldosterone system (RAAS), a complex hormonal pathway that regulates blood pressure. When blood pressure drops, special cells in the kidneys release an enzyme called renin. Renin acts on a protein called angiotensinogen to convert it into angiotensin I. Angiotensin-converting enzyme (ACE), primarily produced by the lungs, converts angiotensin I into angiotensin II. Angiotensin II is a potent vasoconstrictor that narrows blood vessels, raising blood pressure. Aldosterone acts on the kidneys to increase sodium reabsorption, leading to water retention and elevated blood volume, which further raises blood pressure.

Blood Pressure's Impact on Kidney Function:

Maintaining appropriate blood pressure is crucial for kidney health. High blood pressure can damage the delicate blood vessels within the kidneys, impairing their filtration ability and leading to kidney disease. Chronic hypertension can result in hypertensive nephropathy, a condition characterized by progressive kidney damage.

Autoregulation of Kidney Blood Flow:

The kidneys have an autoregulatory mechanism that helps maintain a relatively constant blood flow despite changes in systemic blood pressure. Specialized cells in the kidneys sense changes in pressure and adjust the diameter of the blood vessels to maintain a stable blood flow. This mechanism ensures that the kidneys receive adequate blood supply while avoiding excessive strain due to high blood pressure.

Sodium and Fluid Balance:

The kidneys play a crucial role in regulating sodium (salt) and fluid balance, which directly impacts blood pressure. By adjusting the reabsorption and excretion of sodium, the kidneys influence the body's overall fluid volume. High sodium intake can lead to fluid retention and increased blood volume, raising blood pressure.

Blood Pressure's Influence on Glomerular Filtration Rate (GFR):

The glomerular filtration rate (GFR) is a measure of how effectively the kidneys filter waste and excess substances from the blood. High blood pressure can damage the small blood vessels in the kidneys (glomeruli), reducing their filtration capacity and leading to decreased GFR.

EXPLANATION OF HOW KIDNEY DISEASE CAN LEAD TO HYPERTENSION.

Kidney disease and hypertension (high blood pressure) often go hand in hand in a complex interplay. Kidney disease can both contribute to the development of hypertension and be a consequence of longstanding uncontrolled high blood pressure. This relationship highlights the crucial role of the kidneys in regulating blood pressure and maintaining overall health.

Renal Hypertension:

One common way kidney disease leads to hypertension is through a condition known as renal hypertension or renovascular hypertension. The kidneys play a significant role in regulating blood pressure through the renin-angiotensin-aldosterone system (RAAS). When the kidneys are damaged due to kidney disease, this system can become dysregulated.

RAAS Dysregulation: Kidney damage can disrupt the normal functioning of the RAAS, causing overproduction of renin. This results in elevated levels of angiotensin II, a potent vasoconstrictor. Angiotensin II narrows blood vessels, increases blood volume by stimulating aldosterone production, and triggers the release of antidiuretic hormone (ADH), all of which lead to increased blood pressure.

Fluid Retention: Kidney disease can lead to impaired sodium and fluid balance. When the kidneys can't efficiently excrete excess sodium, the body retains more fluid, increasing blood volume and contributing to higher blood pressure.

Reduced Nitric Oxide Production:

Nitric oxide is a molecule that helps blood vessels relax and dilate, promoting normal blood flow and regulating blood pressure. In kidney disease, reduced nitric oxide production can lead to blood vessel constriction, contributing to hypertension.

Inflammation and Oxidative Stress:

Kidney disease is associated with inflammation and oxidative stress, which can damage blood vessels and impair their ability to relax and contract properly. This can lead to increased resistance in the blood vessels, causing elevated blood pressure.

Reduced Glomerular Filtration Rate (GFR):

As kidney disease progresses, the glomerular filtration rate (GFR), which measures the kidneys' ability to filter waste and excess substances from the blood, decreases. This reduced filtration capacity can lead to the accumulation of substances that can affect blood vessel tone and contribute to hypertension.

Hormonal Imbalances:

Kidney disease can lead to hormonal imbalances, including elevated levels of parathyroid hormone and decreased levels of active vitamin D. These imbalances can affect blood vessel function and contribute to hypertension.

Excessive Sodium Retention:

Damaged kidneys may have difficulty excreting excess sodium, leading to sodium retention in the body. This can result in increased fluid volume and elevated blood pressure.

DISCUSSION OF SYMPTOMS RELATED TO HIGH BLOOD PRESSURE AND ITS POTENTIAL IMPACT ON OVERALL HEALTH.

High blood pressure, also known as hypertension, is often referred to as the "silent killer" because it often doesn't cause noticeable symptoms until it reaches advanced stages. However, untreated high blood pressure can have a significant impact on overall health and increase the risk of serious complications.

SYMPTOMS OF HIGH BLOOD PRESSURE: Most people with high blood pressure do not experience specific symptoms, which is why regular blood pressure monitoring is essential for early detection. However, in some cases, individuals with extremely high blood pressure may experience:

Headaches: Severe headaches, especially in the back of the head, can sometimes be a symptom of extremely high blood pressure. However, headaches are a nonspecific symptom and can have various other causes.

Nosebleeds: In some cases, high blood pressure can lead to nosebleeds. However, nosebleeds are more commonly caused by other factors, such as dry air or nasal irritation.

POTENTIAL IMPACT ON OVERALL
HEALTH:

Cardiovascular System: High blood pressure can damage the blood vessels, leading to atherosclerosis (narrowing and hardening of arteries), increasing the risk of heart attack, stroke, and other cardiovascular diseases.

Brain: Chronic high blood pressure increases the risk of stroke by damaging blood vessels in the brain or causing blood vessel rupture.

Kidneys: Hypertension can damage the kidneys' blood vessels and reduce their ability to filter waste from the blood, potentially leading to chronic kidney disease.

Eyes: High blood pressure can damage the blood vessels in the eyes, leading to vision problems or even blindness in severe cases.

Peripheral Arterial Disease (PAD): Hypertension can contribute to the development of PAD, which affects blood flow to the limbs and increases the risk of infections, ulcers, and amputations.

Metabolic Syndrome: Hypertension is often part of a constellation of metabolic abnormalities that increase the risk of type 2 diabetes and cardiovascular disease.

Overall Quality of Life: Chronic high blood pressure can impact overall well-being, leading to fatigue, reduced physical activity, and increased stress.

THE IMPORTANCE OF MANAGEMENT: Given the potential serious consequences of untreated high blood pressure, early detection and management are crucial. Lifestyle modifications, including a healthy diet, regular exercise, weight management, reduced sodium intake, and stress management, are key components of managing high blood pressure. In some cases, medications may be prescribed to help lower blood pressure.

CHAPTER 7: SYSTEMIC SYMPTOMS AND COMPLICATIONS

EXPLORING SYMPTOMS THAT EXTEND BEYOND THE KIDNEYS: CARDIOVASCULAR ISSUES, FATIGUE, NAUSEA, LOSS OF APPETITE

Symptoms of kidney disease can extend beyond the kidneys and affect various body systems, leading to a range of general and specific manifestations. Here's an exploration of how kidney disease can impact cardiovascular health and contribute to symptoms like fatigue, nausea, and loss of appetite:

Cardiovascular Issues:

Kidney disease can have significant effects on the cardiovascular system due to its impact on fluid balance, electrolyte levels, and blood pressure regulation. Some cardiovascular symptoms associated with kidney disease include:

High Blood Pressure (Hypertension): Kidney disease can disrupt the body's mechanisms for regulating blood pressure, leading to hypertension. Elevated blood pressure puts added strain on the heart and blood vessels, increasing the risk of heart disease, heart attack, and stroke.

Fluid Retention and Edema: Kidney disease can cause fluid retention, leading to swelling in the legs, ankles, and other parts of the body. This can contribute to the development of congestive heart failure and worsen existing cardiovascular conditions.

Increased Risk of Cardiovascular Disease: Chronic kidney disease is associated with an increased risk of atherosclerosis (narrowing and hardening of arteries), heart attack, and other cardiovascular complications.

Fatigue:

Fatigue is a common symptom in individuals with kidney disease. Several factors contribute to this:

Anemia: Kidney disease can lead to reduced production of erythropoietin, a hormone that stimulates red blood cell production. This can result in anemia, which causes fatigue due to decreased oxygen-carrying capacity

THE CONNECTION BETWEEN KIDNEY DISEASE AND WEAKENED IMMUNE SYSTEM, AND RELATED SYMPTOMS

There is a complex and bidirectional relationship between kidney disease and the immune system. Kidney disease can weaken the immune system, making individuals more susceptiblc to infections, while immune system dysfunction can contribute to the development and progression of kidney disease.

Immune System Dysfunction in Kidney Disease: Kidneys play a role in immune system regulation by filtering waste products, metabolites, and immune complexes. Kidney disease can disrupt this balance and lead to immune system dysfunction:

Reduced Immune Response: Chronic kidney disease can suppress the immune response, making individuals more vulnerable to infections. The body's ability to fight off bacteria, viruses, and other pathogens may be compromised.

Increased Inflammation: Kidney disease can lead to chronic inflammation, which can affect immune system function. Inflammation may result from the accumulation of waste products and the activation of inflammatory pathways.

Alteration of Immune Cells: Kidney disease can alter the distribution and function of immune cells, affecting their ability to respond to infections and other immune challenges.

Susceptibility to Infections:

Kidney disease can weaken the immune system's ability to fend off infections, leading to a higher risk of various infections:

Urinary Tract Infections (UTIs): Kidney disease can impair the body's ability to fight off UTIs, which can be more frequent and severe in individuals with compromised kidney function.

Respiratory Infections: Weakened immune responses in kidney disease may increase the risk of respiratory infections such as pneumonia.

Skin Infections: Impaired immune function can also lead to skin infections that are difficult to treat.

Anemia and Immune Function:

Anemia is common in kidney disease due to reduced production of erythropoietin (EPO), a hormone that stimulates red blood cell production. Anemia can impact immune function indirectly:

Reduced Oxygen Delivery: Anemia decreases the oxygen-carrying capacity of the blood, potentially affecting the function of immune cells.

T-Cell Dysfunction: Anemia can impair the function of T cells, which are crucial for adaptive immune responses.

Immunosuppressive Medications:

In cases where kidney disease is treated with immunosuppressive medications (e.g., in kidney transplant recipients), the immune system is intentionally suppressed to prevent the body from rejecting the transplanted kidney. While these medications are necessary, they can increase the risk of infections.

Related Symptoms:

Symptoms related to a weakened immune system in kidney disease can include:

Frequent Infections: Recurrent infections, such as UTIs, respiratory infections, and skin infections, may be a sign of an impaired immune response.

Slow Healing: Wounds or injuries may take longer to heal due to compromised immune function.

Fatigue: Dealing with chronic infections can lead to persistent fatigue and low energy levels.

Unexplained Fever: Frequent or unexplained fever may indicate ongoing infections that the immune system is struggling to control.

Poor Response to Treatment: If infections are challenging to treat or frequently recur, it may suggest an underlying immune system issue.

SKIN-RELATED SYMPTOMS AND THEIR CONNECTION TO KIDNEY DYSFUNCTION

Skin-related symptoms can be indicative of kidney dysfunction, as the kidneys play a crucial role in maintaining overall health and eliminating waste products from the body. Kidney dysfunction can lead to the buildup of waste products and imbalances in electrolytes, which can manifest in various skin-related symptoms.

Uremic Frost:

Uremic frost is a rare but distinctive sign of severe kidney dysfunction. It occurs when urea and other waste products are excreted through the skin, forming white or grayish powdery deposits on the skin's surface. This symptom is often accompanied by other signs of advanced kidney disease, such as fatigue, nausea, and decreased urine output.

Pruritus (Itching):

Persistent and severe itching (pruritus) is a common symptom in individuals with kidney disease, particularly those undergoing dialysis. The exact cause of pruritus in kidney disease is not fully understood, but it is believed to be related to the buildup of toxins and imbalances in minerals like calcium and phosphorus.

Skin Discoloration:

Kidney dysfunction can lead to changes in skin color, including:

Pale or Yellowish Skin: Anemia, common in kidney disease due to reduced red blood cell production, can cause the skin to appear pale. Additionally, a buildup of waste products in the blood can cause the skin to take on a yellowish hue (jaundice).

Gray or Bronze Skin: A condition called "gray skin syndrome" or "bronze diabetes" can occur in advanced kidney disease, leading to a gray or bronze discoloration of the skin, particularly on the face and neck.

Easy Bruising and Bleeding:

Kidney dysfunction can lead to platelet dysfunction and clotting abnormalities, resulting in easy bruising and bleeding. This can manifest as small red or purple spots on the skin (petechiae) or larger bruises.

Edema and Swelling:

Edema, or fluid retention, is a common symptom in kidney disease. While it often affects the legs, ankles, and feet, it can also cause puffiness and swelling in the face, around the eyes, and even in the hands.

Dry and Flaky Skin:

Kidney dysfunction can disrupt the body's fluid and electrolyte balance, potentially leading to dry and flaky skin due to dehydration.

DISCUSSION OF KIDNEY PAIN AND ITS CHARACTERISTICS

Kidney pain, also known as renal pain or flank pain, refers to discomfort or discomfort felt in the area of the kidneys, typically located in the upper back or the sides of the abdomen. It's important to differentiate between true kidney pain and pain originating from other nearby structures, as the underlying causes and implications can vary.

CHARACTERISTICS OF KIDNEY PAIN

Location: Kidney pain is typically felt on one side of the back, below the ribcage. It can radiate to the lower abdomen, groin, and even the thighs. The pain tends to be focused on the area around the kidneys, which are located just below the ribcage on either side of the spine.

Nature of Pain: Kidney pain is often described as a dull ache or throbbing sensation.

Flank Pain: The term "flank pain" is often used to describe kidney pain. Flank refers to the area between the lower ribs and the hip bone.

Pain Triggers: Kidney pain can be worsened by certain movements, such as bending, twisting, or deep breathing. It may also be aggravated by pressure on the area.

Associated Symptoms: Kidney pain is often accompanied by other symptoms, such as urinary changes (blood in urine, changes in frequency or urgency), fever, chills, nausea, vomiting, and pain while urinating.

POSSIBLE CAUSES OF KIDNEY PAIN

Kidney Infections (Pyelonephritis): Infections of the kidneys, often caused by bacteria that travel from the urinary tract, can lead to inflammation and pain.

Kidney Stones: Solid mineral deposits that form in the kidneys can cause intense pain as they move through the urinary tract.

Urinary Tract Obstruction: Blockages in the urinary tract, such as from a kidney stone or enlarged prostate, can lead to pain and discomfort.

Kidney Injury: Trauma or injury to the kidneys can result in pain, especially if the trauma leads to bleeding or inflammation.

Polycystic Kidney Disease: This genetic disorder causes the growth of fluid-filled cysts in the kidneys, leading to pain and discomfort.

Glomerulonephritis: Inflammation of the kidney's filtering units (glomeruli) can cause kidney pain along with other symptoms.

Hydronephrosis: Swelling of the kidney due to urine backup can lead to pain.

DIFFERENTIATING BETWEEN KIDNEY PAIN AND BACK PAIN.

Differentiating between kidney pain and back pain can be challenging because their symptoms can overlap, and the pain may radiate to different areas. However, understanding the characteristics and associated symptoms of each type of pain can help distinguish between them.

Kidney Pain:

Location: Kidney pain is typically felt in the upper back or the sides of the abdomen, just below the ribcage. It often occurs on one side, but if both kidneys are affected, the pain can be bilateral.

Nature of Pain: Kidney pain is often described as a dull ache or throbbing sensation. It can be intermittent or continuous and may come in waves. It's not usually affected by movement.

Radiation: Kidney pain can radiate from the back to the lower abdomen, groin, and even the thighs.

Pain Triggers: Kidney pain might be aggravated by pressure on the affected area, but it's not typically affected by bending, twisting, or deep breathing.

BACK PAIN:

Location: Back pain is usually centered in the lower back, although it can affect any part of the back, including the upper back.

Nature of Pain: Back pain can vary in intensity and may be sharp, dull, or achy. It can be affected by movement and certain positions.

Radiation: Back pain can radiate down the legs, following the path of the nerves. This is known as referred pain and is not typically associated with kidney pain.

Associated Symptoms: Back pain is not typically associated with urinary symptoms like blood in urine, changes in urinary frequency, or pain while urinating. It's also not commonly accompanied by fever or chills unless there's an underlying infection.

Pain Triggers: Back pain can be triggered or worsened by movements, such as bending, twisting, or lifting heavy objects.

EXPLORING THE CONNECTION BETWEEN KIDNEY STONES AND PAIN SYMPTOMS

Certainly, let's delve deeper into the connection between kidney stones and the pain symptoms they can cause:

Formation of Kidney Stones:

Kidney stones, also known as renal calculi, are solid mineral and crystal deposits that form within the kidneys. They can vary in size, from tiny grains to larger, more complex structures. Kidney stones are typically made up of substances like calcium, oxalate, uric acid, and other minerals found in urine.

Pain Characteristics Associated with Kidney Stones:

Flank Pain: One of the hallmark symptoms of kidney stones is flank pain. Flank pain refers to discomfort or pain in the area between the ribcage and the hip, on the side where the affected kidney is located.

Sudden Onset: Kidney stone pain often comes on suddenly and without warning. The pain can escalate rapidly to intense levels.

Colicky Pain: The pain caused by kidney stones is often described as colicky, meaning it comes in waves or episodes of intense discomfort. These waves can last for several minutes to hours.

Intensity: The pain associated with kidney stones is renowned for its intensity. It's often described as excruciating and can be more severe than childbirth for some individuals.

Nausea and Vomiting: The severe pain from kidney stones can trigger nausea and vomiting in some cases.

Urinary Symptoms: Kidney stones can lead to symptoms related to the urinary tract, including frequent urination, urgency, and painful urination.

Factors Influencing Pain Severity:

The pain associated with kidney stones can vary depending on several factors:

Stone Size: Larger stones tend to cause more intense pain, especially when they block the flow of urine.

Stone Location: The pain can be affected by the stone's position within the urinary tract. For instance, stones that move from the kidney to the ureter tend to cause more severe pain as they get stuck along the way.

Obstruction: Pain can become more intense if the stone obstructs the flow of urine, causing pressure to build up in the kidney or urinary tract.

MEDICAL ATTENTION:

If you experience sudden, severe flank pain or any symptoms suggestive of kidney stones, it's important to seek medical attention. A healthcare professional can diagnose the presence of kidney stones through imaging tests like CT scans or ultrasound.

CHAPTER 9: PEDIATRIC AND ELDERLY CONSIDERATIONS

UNIQUE SYMPTOMS OF KIDNEY DISEASE IN CHILDREN AND THE ELDERLY

Kidney disease can affect individuals of all ages, including children and the elderly. While many symptoms of kidney disease are similar across different age groups, there are certain unique considerations and symptoms that may be more prevalent or distinct in children and the elderly:

SYMPTOMS OF KIDNEY DISEASE IN CHILDREN

Growth Issues: Children with kidney disease may experience growth failure or stunted growth. Impaired kidney function can affect the body's ability to process nutrients and produce growth-related hormones.

Blood in Urine (Hematuria): Hematuria can be a symptom of kidney disease in children. It might be detected visually or through microscopic examination of the urine.

High Blood Pressure: Hypertension is a concerning symptom in children that can indicate kidney dysfunction. It might not always present with classic symptoms like in adults.

Swelling: Children with kidney disease might develop swelling in the face, around the eyes, or in the extremities due to fluid retention.

Recurrent Urinary Tract Infections (UTIs): Frequent UTIs can be a sign of underlying kidney issues in children. UTIs might be accompanied by fever, pain while urinating, and irritability.

Delayed Milestones: Infants and young children with kidney disease might experience delays in reaching developmental milestones

Bone and Mineral Disorders: Children with kidney disease can develop bone and mineral disorders due to disturbances in calcium and phosphorus metabolism.

SYMPTOMS OF KIDNEY DISEASE IN THE
ELDERLY:

Fatigue and Weakness: Fatigue and weakness can be symptoms of kidney disease in the elderly. These symptoms can be nonspecific but might be exacerbated by anemia associated with kidney dysfunction.

Loss of Appetite and Weight Loss: Elderly individuals with kidney disease might experience a reduced appetite and unintentional weight loss.

Changes in Urination: Elderly individuals might experience changes in urinary habits, including increased frequency, urgency, or nocturia (frequent nighttime urination).

Cognitive Changes: Advanced kidney disease can lead to cognitive changes, confusion, and difficulty concentrating in elderly individuals.

Fluid Overload: Elderly individuals might be more susceptible to fluid overload due to kidney dysfunction, leading to swelling in the ankles, feet, or legs.

Increased Susceptibility to Medication Side Effects: Elderly individuals often take multiple medications. Kidney dysfunction can affect the clearance of drugs from the body, increasing the risk of medication side effects.

Frailty: Kidney disease can contribute to frailty in the elderly, leading to decreased physical function and increased vulnerability to health issues.

EXPLORING GROWTH AND DEVELOPMENT ISSUES IN PEDIATRIC KIDNEY DISEASE

Growth and development issues are significant concerns in pediatric kidney disease, as proper kidney function is essential for normal growth, bone health, and overall development in children. Kidneys play a crucial role in maintaining the body's fluid and electrolyte balance, regulating blood pressure, and filtering waste products from the blood. When kidney function is compromised, it can have a direct impact on a child's growth and development. Here's an exploration of growth and development issues in pediatric kidney disease:

1. Stunted Growth:

Children with kidney disease may experience growth failure or stunted growth. Several factors contribute to this:

Malnutrition: Impaired kidney function can lead to poor appetite, nausea, and vomiting, which can result in inadequate nutrition.

Nutrient Loss: Kidneys are responsible for excreting waste products and excess nutrients. In kidney disease, nutrient loss can occur, leading to deficiencies that affect growth.

Hormonal Imbalances: Kidney dysfunction can disrupt the balance of growth-related hormones such as growth hormone and insulin-like growth factor 1 (IGF-1), which are essential for proper growth.

2. Delayed Puberty:

Children with advanced kidney disease may experience delayed onset of puberty. Hormonal imbalances and chronic illness can affect the timing of puberty-related changes.

3. Bone and Mineral Disorders:

Kidneys play a vital role in maintaining calcium and phosphorus balance, which is essential for bone health. In pediatric kidney disease:

Mineral Imbalances: Disturbances in calcium, phosphorus, and vitamin D metabolism can lead to weakened bones, fractures, and bone pain.

Renal Osteodystrophy: This term refers to a spectrum of bone changes that can occur due to kidney disease, including osteoporosis and osteomalacia (softening of bones).

4. Anemia:

Anemia, often caused by decreased production of erythropoietin (EPO) in kidney disease, can affect oxygen transport to tissues, leading to fatigue, weakness, and reduced physical activity. Anemia can indirectly impact growth and development by reducing overall energy levels.

5. Cognitive Development:

Kidney disease can affect cognitive development in children, particularly in severe cases:

Uremic Encephalopathy: Uremic toxins that accumulate in the bloodstream due to impaired kidney function can affect brain function and cognitive abilities.

Concentration and Learning: Children with kidney disease might experience difficulties with concentration, memory, and learning.

6. Psychosocial Impact:

Chronic kidney disease can have a psychosocial impact on children, leading to stress, anxiety, and emotional challenges that might indirectly affect growth and development.

7. Medication Effects:

Medications used to manage kidney disease, such as steroids and immunosuppressants, can have side effects that impact growth and development.

AGE-RELATED FACTORS CONTRIBUTING TO KIDNEY PROBLEMS IN THE ELDERLY

Kidney problems become more prevalent with age due to a combination of physiological changes, accumulated exposure to risk factors, and the natural aging process.

1. Reduced Kidney Function:

As people age, their kidney function naturally declines. The number of functioning nephrons (the filtering units of the kidneys) decreases, and blood flow to the kidneys may be reduced. This can lead to a decrease in the glomerular filtration rate (GFR), which indicates how well the kidneys are filtering waste from the blood.

2. Changes in Blood Vessels:

Aging can lead to changes in the blood vessels, including the renal arteries that supply blood to the kidneys. These changes can impact blood flow to the kidneys and contribute to kidney dysfunction.

3. Accumulated Exposure to Risk Factors:

Many risk factors for kidney problems accumulate over time, increasing the likelihood of issues in the elderly. These risk factors include high blood pressure, diabetes, obesity, and cardiovascular disease.

4. Chronic Diseases:

The prevalence of chronic diseases that affect kidney health, such as diabetes and hypertension, tends to increase with age. These conditions can directly damage the kidneys over time.

5. Medication Use:

Elderly individuals often take multiple medications, and some medications can have negative effects on kidney function. Certain drugs may be metabolized more slowly in older adults, leading to potential accumulation and increased risk of kidney damage.

6. Dehydration and Fluid Balance:

The elderly are more prone to dehydration due to changes in fluid balance, reduced thirst sensation, and other factors. Dehydration can strain the kidneys and impair their function.

7. Reduced Immune Function:

As the immune system weakens with age, the kidneys may become more susceptible to infections and inflammatory conditions that can affect their function.

8. Increased Risk of Kidney Stones:

The risk of kidney stones tends to rise with age. Dehydration, dietary factors, and reduced kidney function contribute to stone formation.

9. Protein Accumulation:

Aging kidneys may experience protein accumulation in the filtering units (glomeruli), which can impair their ability to effectively filter waste products.

10. Frailty and Overall Health Status:

Frailty and overall health status can impact kidney health in the elderly. Chronic illnesses and conditions associated with aging can contribute to **kidney dysfunction.**

CHAPTER 10: SEEKING HELP AND DIAGNOSIS

IMPORTANCE OF CONSULTING A HEALTHCARE PROFESSIONAL FOR PROPER DIAGNOSIS

Consulting a healthcare professional for proper diagnosis is essential for a variety of reasons, especially when it comes to health issues like kidney problems.

1. Accurate Diagnosis:

Healthcare professionals have the knowledge, training, and expertise to accurately diagnose your condition. Accurate diagnosis is the foundation for effective treatment and management of kidney problems.

2. Identifying Underlying Causes:

Kidney problems can have various underlying causes, ranging from infections and kidney stones to chronic conditions like diabetes and hypertension. A healthcare professional can perform thorough assessments and tests to identify the specific cause of your symptoms.

3. Differentiating from Other Conditions:

Many symptoms of kidney problems can overlap with those of other health issues. A healthcare professional can differentiate between kidney-related symptoms and symptoms caused by other conditions, ensuring you receive the appropriate care.

4. Early Detection and Treatment:

Early detection of kidney problems is crucial for preventing complications and slowing down disease progression. Timely treatment can make a significant difference in managing kidney diseases effectively.

5. Individualized Treatment Plans:

Healthcare professionals can develop personalized treatment plans tailored to your specific condition, medical history, and lifestyle. These plans take into consideration factors like age, underlying conditions, and medication interactions.

6. Monitoring and Follow-Up:

Regular monitoring and follow-up with a healthcare professional are essential for tracking the progression of kidney problems and adjusting treatment plans as needed. This helps ensure that your condition is effectively managed over time.

7. Avoiding Self-Diagnosis and Misinformation:

The internet is full of medical information, but self-diagnosis based on internet research can be inaccurate and lead to unnecessary anxiety. Healthcare professionals rely on evidence-based medical knowledge and diagnostic tools.

8. Preventing Complications:

Kidney problems can lead to serious complications, such as kidney failure, cardiovascular disease, and other health issues. Proper diagnosis and treatment can help prevent or mitigate these complications.

9. Access to Specialized Care:

Certain kidney conditions may require specialized care from nephrologists or other healthcare specialists. Consulting a healthcare professional ensures you're referred to the appropriate specialists if necessary.

10. Peace of Mind:

Consulting a healthcare professional provides peace of mind, knowing that you're receiving expert guidance and care. You can have confidence in the decisions made for your health and well-being.

EXPLANATION OF DIAGNOSTIC TESTS: BLOOD TESTS, URINE TESTS, IMAGING (ULTRASOUND, MRI, CT SCAN)

Diagnostic tests play a crucial role in identifying and evaluating kidney problems. Different tests provide valuable information about kidney function, structure, and potential issues.

1. Blood Tests:

Serum Creatinine and Blood Urea Nitrogen (BUN): These tests measure waste products (creatinine and urea) in the blood. The estimated glomerular filtration rate (eGFR) is calculated based on these values to assess overall kidney function.

Electrolytes: Blood levels of electrolytes like sodium, potassium, and calcium are assessed. Imbalances in these electrolytes can indicate kidney dysfunction.

Complete Blood Count (CBC): This test assesses red and white blood cells, as well as hemoglobin levels. Anemia due to kidney disease can be detected through CBC results.

Blood Glucose: Elevated blood glucose levels may indicate diabetes, a common cause of kidney problems.

2. Urine Tests:

Urinalysis: This test examines the physical and chemical properties of urine, including color, appearance, pH, protein, glucose, blood cells, and specific gravity. Abnormalities may suggest kidney disease, infection, or other issues.

Urine Protein-to-Creatinine Ratio (PCR) or Albumin-to-Creatinine Ratio (ACR): These ratios assess the amount of protein (albumin) in the urine relative to creatinine. Elevated levels can indicate kidney damage or dysfunction.

3. Imaging Tests:

CT Scan (Computed Tomography): A CT scan provides detailed cross-sectional images of the kidneys. It's especially useful for detecting kidney stones, tumors, and structural abnormalities.

4. Kidney Biopsy:

In certain cases, a kidney biopsy may be performed to obtain a small sample of kidney tissue for examination under a microscope. This helps diagnose specific kidney diseases, assess the extent of damage, and guide treatment decisions.

ENCOURAGING REGULAR HEALTH CHECK-UPS FOR EARLY DETECTION AND PREVENTION

Regular health check-ups are an integral part of maintaining overall well-being and preventing potential health issues. When it comes to kidney health and other medical conditions, early detection and prevention play a significant role in ensuring optimal health outcomes.

1. Early Detection of Kidney Problems:

Regular health check-ups allow healthcare professionals to monitor your kidney function and detect any abnormalities or changes early on. Early detection of kidney problems can lead to timely intervention and management, preventing the progression of kidney disease and potential complications.

2. Preventive Care:

Health check-ups provide an opportunity for healthcare providers to assess your risk factors for kidney disease and other health conditions. Through preventive care, you can receive guidance on lifestyle modifications, such as maintaining a healthy diet, staying physically active, managing blood pressure and blood sugar levels, and avoiding tobacco and excessive alcohol use.

3. Identification of Risk Factors:

Regular health check-ups help identify risk factors that may contribute to kidney problems, such as hypertension, diabetes, obesity, and family history of kidney disease. Addressing these risk factors early can significantly reduce the likelihood of developing kidney issues.

4. Personalized Recommendations:

Health check-ups allow healthcare professionals to provide personalized recommendations based on your individual health status, age, medical history, and lifestyle. These recommendations can help you make informed decisions about your health and well-being.

5. Monitoring Chronic Conditions:

If you have existing chronic conditions like diabetes or hypertension, regular health check-ups enable healthcare providers to closely monitor your kidney health as part of managing these conditions effectively.

6. Preventing Complications:

Detecting and managing kidney problems early can prevent complications such as kidney failure, cardiovascular disease, and related health issues. Early intervention can lead to better quality of life and improved health outcomes.

7. Educating and Empowering Individuals:
Health check-ups offer opportunities for healthcare providers to educate individuals about kidney health, the importance of hydration, signs of potential kidney problems, and how to take proactive steps to maintain kidney health.

8. Reducing Healthcare Costs:
Preventive care through regular health check-ups can help identify and address health issues at an early stage, reducing the need for more intensive and costly medical interventions later.

CHAPTER 11: MANAGEMENT AND LIFESTYLE CHANGES

LIFESTYLE MODIFICATIONS TO SUPPORT KIDNEY HEALTH: DIETARY ADJUSTMENTS, HYDRATION, EXERCISE

Lifestyle modifications play a crucial role in supporting kidney health and reducing the risk of kidney problems. Making positive changes to your diet, staying hydrated, and incorporating regular exercise can have a significant impact on kidney function and overall well-being.

1. Dietary Adjustments:

Monitor Sodium Intake: Reduce your sodium (salt) intake, as excess sodium can lead to high blood pressure and fluid retention. Choose fresh, unprocessed foods, and limit the use of salt in cooking and at the table.

Control Protein Intake: While protein is essential, excessive protein consumption can strain the kidneys. Consume a moderate amount of high-quality protein sources, such as lean meats, fish, poultry, eggs, and plant-based proteins.

Limit Phosphorus and Potassium: If you have kidney problems, limit foods high in phosphorus (dairy products, nuts, seeds) and potassium (bananas, oranges, potatoes) to avoid mineral imbalances.

Choose Healthy Fats: Opt for healthy fats from sources like olive oil, avocados, and nuts. Limit saturated and trans fats found in fried and processed foods.

Stay Hydrated: Drink plenty of water throughout the day to help maintain proper kidney function and prevent dehydration. Adequate hydration supports kidney filtration and helps prevent kidney stone formation.

Reduce Sugar Intake: Minimize consumption of sugary foods and beverages, which can contribute to diabetes and obesity, both of which are risk factors for kidney problems.

Monitor Phosphate Additives: Processed foods often contain phosphate additives that can negatively impact kidney health. Read labels and avoid products with high phosphate content.

2. Hydration:

Drink Water Regularly: Staying adequately hydrated is essential for kidney health. Aim to drink water throughout the day and adjust your intake based on factors like activity level and weather.

3. Exercise:

Engage in Regular Physical Activity: Exercise helps maintain a healthy weight, supports cardiovascular health, and improves overall well-being. Aim for at least 150 minutes of moderate-intensity aerobic activity or 75 minutes of vigorous activity per week, as recommended by health guidelines.

Consult Your Healthcare Provider: If you have existing kidney problems, consult your healthcare provider before starting a new exercise routine.

They can provide guidance on suitable activities and intensity levels.

4. Lifestyle Factors:

Manage Blood Pressure and Blood Sugar: High blood pressure and diabetes are leading causes of kidney problems. Regularly monitor your blood pressure and blood sugar levels, and follow your healthcare provider's recommendations for managing these conditions.

Avoid Smoking and Limit Alcohol: Smoking and excessive alcohol consumption can harm kidney function and contribute to various health issues. Quit smoking and limit alcohol intake to support your kidneys and overall health.

Get Enough Sleep: Prioritize quality sleep, as adequate rest supports overall health and immune function.

MEDICATION MANAGEMENT AND ADHERENCE

Medication management and adherence are essential components of maintaining kidney health, managing kidney problems, and preventing complications. Properly taking prescribed medications as directed by your healthcare provider can significantly impact the progression of kidney disease and overall well-being.

1. Understand Your Medications:

Know Your Medications: Understand the names, purposes, dosages, and potential side effects of the medications you're taking.

2. Communicate with Healthcare Providers:

Regular Follow-Ups: Attend scheduled appointments with your healthcare provider to discuss your medications, monitor your kidney health, and adjust your treatment plan as needed.

Inform Your Healthcare Provider: Keep your healthcare provider informed about all the medications, supplements, and over-the-counter drugs you're taking to avoid potential interactions.

3. Medication Adherence:

Follow Prescribed Instructions: Take medications exactly as prescribed by your healthcare provider. Follow the recommended dosage, frequency, and timing.

Use Pill Organizers: Pill organizers can help you keep track of daily doses, reducing the risk of missed doses or accidental double doses.

Set Reminders: Use alarms, phone apps, or written reminders to help you remember to take your medications on time.

Incorporate into Routine: Align your medication schedule with daily routines, such as meals or bedtime, to help make adherence easier.

Travel Considerations: If you're traveling, ensure you have enough medication for the duration of your trip, and keep medications in their original packaging.

4. Over-the-Counter Medications and Supplements:

Consult Your Healthcare Provider: Before taking any over-the-counter medications, herbal supplements, or vitamins, consult your healthcare provider to ensure they won't negatively impact your kidney health or interact with prescribed medications.

5. Medication Side Effects:

Monitor Side Effects: Be aware of potential side effects of your medications. If you experience any unusual symptoms, notify your healthcare provider promptly.

6. Storage and Disposal:

Proper Storage: Store medications as instructed on the packaging, in a cool, dry place, away from direct sunlight and moisture.

Disposal: Dispose of expired or unused medications properly according to local guidelines.

7. Team Approach:

Pharmacist Support: Consult your pharmacist if you have questions about your medications, including potential interactions or side effects.

Engage Family Members: If needed, involve family members or caregivers to help you manage your medications and adhere to your treatment plan.

WHEN AND HOW TO CONSIDER MEDICAL INTERVENTIONS LIKE DIALYSIS OR TRANSPLANTATION

Medical interventions like dialysis and kidney transplantation are considered when kidney function becomes significantly impaired, leading to complications and reduced quality of life. Decisions regarding these interventions are made in collaboration with healthcare providers and are based on various factors.

Dialysis:

Dialysis is a medical procedure that involves filtering waste products and excess fluids from the blood when the kidneys can no longer perform this function effectively. It's typically considered when:

End-Stage Renal Disease (ESRD): Dialysis is often recommended for individuals with ESRD, which is the final stage of kidney disease where kidney function is severely compromised (eGFR < 15 mL/min/1.73 m^2).

Symptoms and Complications: Dialysis may be necessary when kidney disease leads to symptoms such as severe fatigue, nausea, vomiting, fluid overload, electrolyte imbalances, and high levels of waste products in the blood.

Inability to Maintain Balance: When the kidneys cannot maintain proper fluid and electrolyte balance, and these imbalances pose a risk to health, dialysis becomes crucial.

Kidney Transplantation:

Kidney transplantation involves replacing a damaged kidney with a healthy kidney from a donor. It's considered when:

ESRD and Reduced Quality of Life: For individuals with ESRD, a kidney transplant offers the opportunity for improved quality of life compared to long-term dialysis.

Suitable Donor Available: A suitable living or deceased donor is identified. The donor's blood type and tissue compatibility are matched to minimize the risk of organ rejection.

Age and Health Status: The recipient's age, overall health, and ability to tolerate surgery and immunosuppressive medications are assessed. Comprehensive Evaluation: Both the recipient and donor undergo thorough medical, psychological, and compatibility evaluations to ensure a successful transplant.

Factors to Consider:

Quality of Life: Both dialysis and transplantation can significantly improve quality of life for individuals with kidney problems.

Long-Term Commitment: Transplant recipients require lifelong immunosuppressive medications to prevent organ rejection. Dialysis requires regular sessions and lifestyle adjustments.

Medical Evaluation: Consult nephrologists, transplant specialists, and healthcare providers to discuss your individual situation, options, risks, benefits, and expected outcomes.

The Fertility Factor

A Step-by-Step Guide to Achieving Your Family Dreams

Rossana Lewis